Wade Minor Logan

Consumption

It's Pathology and Treatment

Wade Minor Logan

Consumption
It's Pathology and Treatment

ISBN/EAN: 9783744669931

Printed in Europe, USA, Canada, Australia, Japan

Cover: Foto ©Andreas Hilbeck / pixelio.de

More available books at **www.hansebooks.com**

CONSUMPTION:

ITS

PATHOLOGY AND TREATMENT.

TO WHICH IS APPENDED

AN ESSAY ON THE USE OF ALCOHOL

IN THE

TREATMENT OF CONSUMPTION.

BY WADE MINOR LOGAN, M.D.

—

S. W. BUTLER, M.D., PHILADELPHIA.

1871.

PREFACE.

My object in offering this little work to my professional brethren is simply to afford them the results of some observations made, and conclusions arrived at, in regard to the Pathology and Treatment of Tubercular Consumption, especially touching Nitric Acid as a remedial agent in combating "that fell disease." I hope, however, not to be understood as claiming to have found a specific. I am, nevertheless, confident that in nitric acid we have an invaluable remedy. If this monograph shall inspire sufficient confidence in the views expressed to induce a fair and full trial of the plan of treatment here recommended, I am perfectly willing to abide the verdict of experience as to its virtue. It being my object to present only the results of my own researches and investigations, presuming the professional reader to be familiar with standard authorities and treatises on this subject, including especially Physical Diagnosis, Hygienics, Climatology, etc., little or nothing is said on those subjects. Neither would it be appropriate to attempt here a discussion of the commonly-received opinions as to the Etiology, Pathology and Treatment of Consumption. As before stated, they are only presented wherein I have original views to offer.

In Chapter IV, liberal quotations are made from CAR-PENTER's "Prize Essay on Alcoholic Liquors," as apology for which I cannot do better than cite the following language of DICKENS in his introductory paragraph to the "Pickwick Papers":—"Many authors entertain not only a foolish, but a really dishonest objection to acknowledge the sources from whence they derive much valuable information. We have no such feeling. . . . Whatever ambition we might have felt under other circumstances to lay claim to the authorship of these" opinions, "a regard for truth forbids us to do more than claim the merit of their judicious arrangement and impartial narration. . . . . . . The labors of others have raised for us an immense reservoir of important facts," which I have used so far as available, feeling grateful that such facts and observations not only sustained my own views, but coming from the eminent source which they do, renders them doubly authoritative on the subject under consideration. It may be said, by way of objection, by those who may not coincide in my views, that the Prize Essay of Dr. CAR-

PENTER, of which comparatively liberal use has been made in the preparation of the chapter on Alcohol in Consumption, has reference to the effects of alcoholic liquors on the healthy human system; but Prof. CHAMBERS,* of London, says: "The best guide to the effects to be expected from a re-agent on a diseased body is the intelligent observation of its effects on a healthy body; and I think that alcohol is no exception, but that a knowledge of its physiological action leads directly to its therapeutical application." The views given in this chapter are so opposed to those generally entertained by medical men, that I cannot hope for them to escape severe criticism; nevertheless, they announce my candid convictions on a subject of great importance, and I humbly send them forth, hoping that good may result therefrom.

W. M. L.

Cincinnati, December, 1871.

* Renewal of Life, p. 605.

CONTENTS.

CHAPTER I:

PATHOLOGY OF CONSUMPTION.

Investigations of the Author.—Chemical Analysis of Tubercle.—Phosphate of Lime in.—Condition of Costal Cartilages in Tuberculosis.—Abundance of Phosphates in Food.—Gray Tubercle, General Character of.—Cretaceous Tubercle.—Origin of Tuberculosis.—Mode of Deposit of Tubercles.—Transformation of Gray into Yellow Tubercle.—Mode of Transformation.—Softening of Tubercles.—Condition of Blood Plasma.—Fatty Liver.

CHAPTER II.

ETIOLOGY OF CONSUMPTION.

Influences Causing Consumption.—Predisposition to the Disease, both Inherited and Acquired.—Effects of want of Food and Air.—Mode in which Sedentary Life and Deficient Ventilation Cause Consumption.—Frequency of Development of Secondary Tuberculosis in Phthisical Lungs.—Chemical Action of Fresh Air (its oxygen) for the Prevention of Consumption.—How " Chronic Pneumonia" may cause Tuberculosis.—Comparative Infrequency of Formation of Cavities from " Caseous Infiltration."

(vii)

CHAPTER III.

TREATMENT OF CONSUMPTION.

Nitric and Muriatic Acids, Medical Properties of.—Use of Nitric Acid in Whooping Cough, Chronic Bronchitis, and Hoarseness of Singers.—In the Healing of Phagadenic and Flabby Ulcers.—For the Solution of Phosphatic Calculi.—Rationale of the Action of Nitric Acid.—Muriatic Acid, its Properties and Mode of Action.—Digestive Assimilation of Medicine.—Mode of Administering the Acids.—Cases Reported.—Removal of Tubercles from the Lungs.

CHAPTER IV.

ALCOHOL IN CONSUMPTION.

Effects of Alcoholic Liquors on the Solids and Fluids of the Body—On the Plasma and Nutrition—As a Retarder of both *Destructive* and *Constructive* Metamorphosis of Tissue.—Effects of Deficient Plasticity of the Blood.—*Apparent* Robustness Produced by the Ingestion of Alcohol Fallacious.—Bad Effects of Alcohol on the Nutrition of the Nervous System.—Alcohol an Arrester of Nerve Life.—Amblyopia (impaired vision) Superinduced by "Chronic, *not Excessive*, use of Alcoholic Drinks.—Influence of the Nervous System on Nutrition.—Examples where Deficient.—Alcohol a Diminisher of Nerve Force.—Supposed uses of Alcohol.—Transientness of the Effects of Stimulants.—Fallacy of their Usual Employment.—Use of Alcohol in Exceptional Cases.—Alcohol Destructive to Pepsin.—Medicines Employed in its Stead.—Effects of Alcohol on Inflammation.—Physiological *modus operandi* of Alcoholic Stimulants.—*How Alcohol does Positive Damage to the Lungs.*—The Author's Conclusions.

CONSUMPTION:

ITS

PATHOLOGY AND TREATMENT.

CHAPTER I.

PATHOLOGY OF TUBERCULAR CONSUMPTION.

Without pausing to discuss the relative merits of the various theories that have been proposed concerning the nature of this disease, or for other preliminaries, I proceed to the consideration of some investigations that I have recently made.

The chemical analysis of tubercle shows that the phosphates, especially the phosphate of lime is the inorganic element of this morbid deposit, just as iron is an inorganic element of hæmatin. And according to that law of physiological chemistry known as vital affinity, we would reasonably expect the introduction of the phosphates into the system of a tuberculous subject to give rise to a corresponding increase of the tubercular deposit. And by a

1 (9)

series of experiments conducted by Mr. JOHN TAYLOR* upon tuberculous subjects in the Liverpool workhouse, they were found to hasten the development of the disease; and would, therefore, seem to tend conclusively, in the estimation of that gentleman, to the establishment of our hypothesis.

Such distinguished men as Profs. L. M. LAWSON, GEORGE B. WOOD, and HENRY HARTSHORNE, and Drs. COTTON, QUAIN, J. R. BENNETT, and M. DECHAMBRE, of Paris, after repeated trial of the phosphates and hypophosphites of lime, soda, and potassa, have published the results of their experiments, expressing their discouragement.

I do not know of any one who now claims for them that degree of reputation which Drs. STONE, CHURCHILL, and others, at one time anticipated they would enjoy. I have, indeed, been employed in cases in which the patient had gradually sunk under them in the care of other and first-class practitioners, when a directly opposite course of medication was instituted, followed by the most flattering results.

" The urine of tuberculous subjects," says LAWSON, " appears to contain less solid constituents, particularly the nitrogenized elements, while the salts, especially the phosphates, are in excess."† This statement has been supported by the majority of my own observations. NIEMEYER, in

* Stillé's Materia Medica, vol. i, Art. Phosphorus, p. 686.
† Lawson's Treatise, p. 454.

speaking of laryngeal phthisis, says, that in the progress of the disease, the laryngeal cartilages frequently undergo ossification. He also states, as do all others, that " it is exceptional for persons deformed by rachitis" (in whose systems there is a deficiency of the phosphates) " to become or die tuberculous."*   "FREUND, of Breslau, regarded ossification of the first costal cartilage as a cause of phthisis, on the hypothesis that it prevented the free expansion of the chest, and by acting as an irritant produced inflammation at the apices."† When a student, long before the conception of this theory, I noticed in opening the chests of a number of tuberculous cadavers, that *all* the costal cartilages were quite hard; one case in particular, a young female apparently about twenty years of age, in one of whose lungs were large tubercular masses, while in the other was a large cavity, and whose costal cartilages were almost as hard as bone, which I then attributed to the disturbance of circulation and nutrition as having probably given rise to an almost perfect state of dryness in those tissues. The "greater prevalence of consumption among the poor than among the more well-to-do classes," NIEMEYER attributes to the food of the former being "chiefly vegetable," and this, it is well known, is the principal source of the element now under consideration.‡

"In ordinary food, there is more of the phosphates than

* Niemeyer's Practice, 7th American Ed., vol. i, p. 129.
† Dr. J. T. Whittaker.
‡ See Niemeyer's Practice, 7th American Ed., vol. i, p. 213.

the system has need of; and in those very disorders in which they are supposed to be indicated, they are not unfrequently in excess in the blood and urine."*

Dr. HEBERDEN paid great attention to this subject, and insists upon the paramount importance of the purity of water, and even went so far as to recommend the use of distilled water. He observed that water loaded with lime proved extremely pernicious. And a striking coincidence is furnished by M. WANNER, of France, who observed that in certain parts of the province of Sologne where the vegetable mold is very shallow and contains no trace of lime, neither consumption nor calculous diseases prevail.†
I would also add, that the use of hard water, especially by consumptives or persons predisposed to consumption, is now seriously objected to by all intelligent physicians, prominently among whom are Drs. HENRY HARTSHORNE and B. W. RICHARDSON. Dr. FRICK, of Baltimore, analyzed the blood of four cases during the existence of *crude* tubercles, and states that, among other deviations from the normal standard, he detected an increase of lime, the quantities in the different cases being respectively .272, .257, .276, .283; remarkably contrasting with .183, the normal proportion: and BAUMES claims to have detected in the blood of tuberculous subjects an excess of phosphoric acid.‡

Again, bearing on this point, Dr. LAWSON, in treating of

* U. S. Dispensatory, 11th Ed., p. 968.
† See Lawson's Treatise on Consumption, p. 274.
‡ Lawson's Treatise on Consumption, pp. 57 and 145.

gray tubercles, says, "they vary in size from that of a
millet seed to that of a pea; and in consistence from a soft
structure *to almost cartilaginous hardness;* being somewhat friable, and presenting a granular surface when cut."*

It is obvious that their soft structure is most probably
due to the deposit being quite recent, still in a partial
state of solution, their more fluid constituents not yet having been absorbed; and that "their *almost cartilaginous
hardness*" is due to their being to a great extent of a calcareous nature, with their fluid properties completely
absorbed.

In regard to cretaceous tubercle, Dr. LAWSON says "the
chemical analysis of cretaceous tubercle shows that the
animal matter becomes absorbed, while the earthy or inorganic materials remain. The relative proportion of the
organic and inorganic substances in the two forms of
tubercle becomes exactly reversed when the cretaceous
change occurs, which is doubtless due to the absorption of
the organic, while the vessels are incapable of taking up
the inorganic. Pathologists speak of this change as absorption of the organic elements, while the deposition of the
inorganic continues, and thus replaces the former substance. According to this view, the earthy material is an
independent secretion, continuing after the deposit of the
ordinary tubercular matter has ceased. It is far more
probable, however, that *the whole mass is deposited in the*

* Lawson's Treatise, pp. 32 and 33.

usual form and composition of tubercle, [italics ours] and that the ulterior changes result from the absorption of the fluid elements, while the earthy substance, being incapable of re-entering the vessels, remains in the cavity."*

Thus it is seen that the phosphates, especially the phosphate of lime, perform no insignificant part in the process of tuberculization and development of phthisis.

Now, in regard to the origin of tuberculosis, let us draw a parallel, by which may be seen the most striking analogy. Sugar normally exists in the blood nowhere else than in the venous circulation between the liver and lungs. In the lungs it is destroyed by the catalytic action of the air; being converted, first, into water; second, into lactic acid; third, into carbonic acid; then and there being voided by the respiratory process.†

Now, if from some defect in elaboration (as often occurs in persons possessing the rheumatic diathesis,) the third change, by which the lactic acid should be converted into carbonic acid, does not take place, blood poisoning would soon be manifested by symptoms of acute articular rheumatism.

So may it not also seem probable‡ that the phosphates,

* Lawson's Treatise, p. 96.
† Williams' Principles of Medicine, p. 163.
‡ "When the *sabulous* deposit" (that is, the phosphates in the urine) "depends upon certain disordered states of digestion, this agent may prove beneficial by restoring the tone of the stomach." (U. S. Dispensatory, 11th Ed., p. 47.)
The "normal change" alluded to in the above paragraph, Prof. Bartholow considers to be that of oxydation.
The eminent authority of Sir Thomas Watson, makes it seem probable

to a certain extent, normally undergo some catalytic or other change, either preparatory to performing or after having performed their function in the economy, and that in the presence of the tuberculous diathesis, by this physiological process being interfered with, either by pre-existing debilitating causes or otherwise, a state of cachexia or blood-poisoning is produced, which, failing to be eliminated from the system, increases in quantity until finally its existence becomes manifested by the familiar phenomena which accompany the development of tuberculosis.

Concerning the deposition of tubercles, the theory accepted by LAWSON, WATSON, and others, was, that it took place by the exudation of a certain specific humor (by us supposed to be to a great extent of a calcareous nature); and Prof. J. H. BENNETT says that "calcareous deposits which do not assume the form of a bony growth are usually the result of an exudation."†

According to the accepted theory on tuberculosis proper, two separate and distinct forms of tubercle were recog-

that besides the oxydation of the phosphates just mentioned, the spleen —although its physiology, and therefore, its pathology, is as yet by no means perfectly understood, so that we can only surmise as to its influence in this respect—performs an important part in the formation of tubercular matter, perhaps by causing further changes in the unoxydized materials. Dr. Watson in regard to tubercular matter, says :

" It is even to be seen sometimes in the blood itself: not indeed while yet contained in its proper vessels, but when it is collected in the cells of the spleen. The spongy texture of that organ allows the blood to accumulate in it in considerable quantity: and the tubercular matter may be seen forming in the blood at some distance from the walls of the cells in which the blood is contained." (Watson's Practice of Physic, by Condie. 1858, p. 149.)

† Bennett's Practice, 3d ed., p. 271.

nized, viz., the gray and the yellow. In regard to the ultimate tendency or result of the two varieties, Dr. LAW-SON says : "While the yellow variety naturally tends to softening and elimination, the gray as constantly under-goes a retrogressive action, and never softens except as a result of its *possible transformation** into the former species," †

How could the gray become transformed into the yellow variety? By acting as a foreign body it would cause in-flammation, and the *consequent exudation* would be in the immediate vicinity of and around the mechanical irritant, and as the more fluid constituents of the exudation would be becoming absorbed by the surrounding lung tissue, its more plastic or solid elements would accumulate around and adhere to the gray tubercle previously deposited, thus transforming the gray into the yellow variety. And we can thus easily understand why yellow tubercle contains a preponderance of albuminous or albuminoid material over either the gray or cretaceous varieties.

And the degraded condition of the blood plasma, pre-sently to be alluded to, which would furnish the exudation with corpuscular rather than coagulable lymph, and whose tendency is to degeneration, explains in my opinion the source of the caseous matter of crude tubercles. Then,

---

* "Læunnec accepted this conversion, which Rokitansky for a long time denied, but now considers frequent. Hérard declares it to be uni-versal." (Hartshorne's Essentials, 2d ed., note at bottom of p. 33.)

† Lawson's Treatise, p. 34.

my opinion is, that after the tubercular exudation, or the exudation of the " *sui generis* specific humor," gray tubercle is the initial lesion of tuberculosis just as chancre is the initial lesion of syphilis.

Thus far I have explained the probable *modus operandi* of tuberculization, that is, the production of a specific humor, which became deposited in the form of a semi-fluid exudation, its development into gray tubercle, which afterward became transformed into yellow tubercle, and this (if not destroyed by suppuration and softening), as a curative agency, into cretaceous tubercle.

SOFTENING OF TUBERCLES.

In an article contributed to the *Medical and Surgical Reporter* last year, I expressed the opinion that this process is " purely suppurative, and an effort of nature to rid herself of the abnormal deposit, just as thorns and other foreign bodies are removed from the flesh by festering." The views of Sir THOMAS WATSON on this subject are expressed in such a clear and beautiful style, and so fully accord with my own, that I cannot do better than quote him. He says: " ANDRAL ascribes the softening of tubercles, not to any spontaneous changes in their central parts, but to the admixture of pus, poured out by the textures immediately surrounding the tubercle which has irritated and inflamed those textures as any other foreign body might.

2

And this statement is nearer the truth than that of LÆN-
NEC, who supposed that crude tubercles after an indefinite
length of time began to soften at their centres." " But you
sometimes find large masses of turbercular matter in the
lungs or elsewhere : and in these masses you see that the
process of softening is going on at several points within
the mass at the same time.   How is this to be explained?
Why these large masses are formed, in fact, by the aggre-
gation of many smaller masses, which, lying near each
other have coalesced as the deposit continued to increase:
and the areolar and other tissues originally intervening
between these coalescing masses at length suppurate; and
by their suppuration, they soften, and gradually break
down the tubercular matter which they enclose, and by
which they are also enclosed.   This is just the process by
which tubercles are frequently expelled from the body.
They increase till the surrounding parts take on inflammation, just as they might do if any foreign body exercised
the same degree of pressure upon them. . . . . . .; the
thin pus which is thrown out pervades and loosens the
tubercular matter; a process of ulceration goes on in the
surrounding textures; and at length (supposing the lung
to have been the seat of the disease) the detritus of the
tubercle is brought up, gradually, by coughing."*

Having considered the four stages of the development of
tubercle, we may mention two frequent, indeed almost

* Watson's Practice of Physic, pp. 149 and 150.

constant concomitants of this disease, viz., the pathological or aplastic condition of the blood plasma, and fatty degeneration of the liver, which, as will hereafter be seen, have a special relation to our method of therapeutics. "Fibrine, identical with the buffy coat of the blood, is the material of which new membranes and cicatrices are formed; it is the *coagulable lymph*, indeed, which is the plasma or basis of the constructive and reparative process. In its capacity for these processes fibrine exhibits some modifications of condition constituting degrees of plasticity. Thus, in a healthy state (euplastic) it forms a fine congeries of minute fibrils, which, having a high capacity for life, may become organized in a high degree, as in the case of false membranes resulting from acute inflammation in a healthy subject. But in many instances, this high capacity is degraded, and the nutritive material is *cacoplastic*, with fewer and less perfect fibres, and with more corpuscles, giving the exudation more opacity, and is susceptible of only a low degree of organization, as in the indurations resulting from low or chronic inflammation, in cirrhosis, gray tubercle, etc.; or it is *aplastic*, not organizable at all, abounding in degenerating corpuscles with few or no fibres, as in pus, curdy matter, yellow tubercle, etc." "In case of deficiency of fibrine from the presence of a febriferous or putrescent poison in the system, it is not to be expected that azotized food, rest, or any other means, can remove the deficiency so long as the poison remains in active operation. This poison, by its septic or other analogous influence, interferes with the vital process by which the fibrine is formed. But no sooner does the influence of the poison subside, as evinced by improvement in the symptoms, than the quantity of the fibrine increases, and this faster than could be explained by any increase of nourishment taken."*

Fatty liver, also, is almost peculiar to phthisis. In three years LOUIS met with it forty-nine times, and forty-seven of the patients died phthisical. It occurred in one-third of the victims of consumption, whereas, among 223 cases not phthisical, there were only two examples of this hepatic change.

* Williams' Principles of Medicine, pp. 157 and 160.

CHAPTER II.

Our limited space and the general plan of this work do not justify us in entering minutely into detail as to the various causes of consumption; even if we believed ourselves competent to thoroughly settle all questions involved in such a discussion, which we do not. This field of investigation has employed the ablest talent of the profession, nevertheless it must be confessed that much remains unknown, and much disagreement exists in the opinions of equally competent writers.

In our chapter on the pathology of consumption we said that it took place in persons having the tuberculous diathesis or predisposition, just as rheumatism and other affections occur in persons having the respective diatheses predisposing to those various affections. As is well known, and in common with other diatheses, the one predisposing to consumption is both inherited and acquired. If at time of begetting the offspring either or both of the parents were consumptive, as NIEMEYER logically says, the diathesis would be "congenital." But we do not agree with him in the opinion that this is the only circumstance under which

(21)

the disease may be considered as inherited. The children of persons whose parents are known to have had tuberculosis are more particularly prone to that disease than to any other;—*peculiarly so*—just as persons having the diathesis predisposing to any other disease are more particularly liable to be attacked with that disease, under the influence of exciting causes, than one toward which they have no such diathetic tendency. As a general principle, to which there are some palpable exceptions,* however, all influences which in the language of NIEMEYER, "retard or disturb the normal development and conservation of the organism" tend to superinduce a predisposition to consumption.

Suppose now that a person in whose parental ancestry there was no trace of tubercular disease or predisposition, during infancy be artificially nourished with diluted cow's or goat's milk, or the more unwholesome milk of an unhealthy wet-nurse, pap, and other unsuitable articles, instead of the mother's milk for which nature at this period makes imperative demand, or that the parents were broken down by debauchery or syphilis, or that there was too great a disparity in the ages and incongruity of the temperaments and habits or nearness of relationship of parents, mental despondency of the mother during gestation and lactation, all or any of which may "retard or disturb the normal development of the organism" and engender a

* The reader is referred to Prof. Lawson's Treatise for authority concerning the immunity afforded consumption by malaria and cancer.

predisposition to the disease,—the predisposition thus entailed upon the progeny would unquestionably be inherited, for if it were not for the pernicious influences mentioned, *cateris paribus,* "the normal development of the organism" would not have been "retarded or disturbed," and *a healthy constitution would have been inherited* instead of a tuberculous diathesis or predisposition to consumption.

But some persons whose parents were perfectly healthy, and who never labored under or were not surrounded by any of the circumstances mentioned, become tuberculous and die phthisical. In this instance the tuberculous diathesis becomes *acquired,* just as the rheumatic and other diatheses sometimes become acquired, when not inherited.

Sedentary habits with insufficient physical exercise, excessive and protracted exertion of either mind or body with a consequent deficiency of repose, intemperance, sexual excesses, syphilitic disease, external influences such as climate with its peculiarities of soil, water, etc., exposure to inclement weather or draughts of air when not properly protected, improper quality or inadequate quantity of food, chronic inflammatory affections of the respiratory organs, and other and even more obscure influences operating either singly or combined in such a manner as to interfere with the chemical, catalytic, molecular, and other changes in the body, thus "retarding or disturbing the normal conservation of the organism" may, and as is well known do frequently induce a predisposition to consumption in persons previously healthy.

As to the relative importance of some of the various influences operating on the system for the production of tubercular consumption, we most fully indorse the following opinions of the late Prof. FELIX VON NIEMEYER, of the University of Tübingen : " Among the influences by which a liability to consumption is acquired, or by which a congenital predisposition to it is aggravated, that of an insufficient or improper diet stands first."* On the same page he says: "The influence of want of fresh air is quite as baneful as is that of an insufficient or improper supply of nourishment. *We have no satisfactory explanation* [italics ours,—see following explanation] *of the mode* in which continuous sedentary life and especially an abode in a close atmosphere charged with effluvia, produces its pernicious effect upon the organism; but the fact has long been established that both scrofula and consumption are far more common in asylums for foundlings and for orphans, in houses of correction, prisons, and among factory operatives who spend the entire day at work in a close room, than among persons who take much exercise in the open air. The objection, that the prevalence of scrofula and consumption in such institutions pro-

* Niemeyer's Text-Book of Practical Medicine, 7th Ed., Vol 1st., p. 213.

ceeds from other causes than lack of fresh air, is untenable. The average diet of the populations of many poor villages is much worse, and the number of prejudicial influences far greater, than is the case among the occupants of prisons and houses of correction, and yet they are not equally subject to these diseases."

Again, our author says that, "exclusive of tuberculosis of the bronchial mucous membrane, the development of secondary tuberculosis in phthisical lungs is of very frequent occurrence." And again he says: "We have no hesitation in stating that the greatest danger, for the majority of consumptives, is, *that they are apt to become tuberculous.* The conditions which cause tuberculosis to accompany many cases of caseous infiltration with formation of cavities * * * *are* [italics ours] *at present unknown to us."* * As Prof. Niemeyer in the foregoing statements frankly acknowledges that he is uninformed as regards the peculiar mode in which the influences there referred to operate to cause tuberculosis, we will venture to offer what we conceive to be a reasonable explanation of this pathological process.

Every medical man is familiar with the importance, indeed, the indispensability of oxygen to the normal performance of the various vital processes, prominently among which are the molecular changes of the body; and the beneficial influence of exercise in the open air (for the pur-

* Same volume as referred to before, pp. 215 and 219.

pose of being benefitted by its oxygen) which is *universally* recommended, especially for consumptives, as well as the well known fact that the more capacity the lungs have for the absorption of oxygen the less is the liability of the organism to become invaded by tuberculosis and perish with the retrogressive action of consumption, affords support to our hypothesis of the oxydation of the phosphates. And as the blood plasma, the function and pathological condition of which we have elsewhere considered, is normally a deutoxide of protein, formed by the action of oxygen upon the protcinaceous constituents of the chyle, and therefore requires for its perfect elaboration an atmosphere rich in oxygen,—"continuous sedentary life, and especially an abode in a close atmosphere charged with effluvia, produces its pernicious effect upon the organism;" and chronic inflammatory affections of the respiratory organs, whether eventuating in "caseous metamorphosis" of the inflammatory product, or otherwise, "cause tuberculosis to accompany many cases of caseous infiltration"— in the former instance by the atmosphere inhaled being deficient in oxygen, in the latter by the pathological condition present interfering with the respiratory process, thus preventing or retarding the normal amount of oxygen from being taken into the system, thereby rendering the pabulum formed, as in case of "insufficient or improper diet," *aplastic*, and inadequate to healthy nutrition, as we have before shown.

Thus we explain how "chronic pneumonia," whether followed by "caseous infiltration" or not, may cause tuberculosis and progressive emaciation of the body, and ultimately tuberculo-inflammatory destruction of the lungs.

Besides hoping that we may have shed an appreciable ray upon the point which we have just been endeavoring to explain, we reproduce the preceding statements, and the one following, from Prof. NIEMEYER, for the purpose of correcting the erroneous inference which many physicians with whom we have conversed seem to have drawn as to its frequency, from his explanation of the destruction of the lungs, and formation of cavities from caseous infiltration, which, as he says, "only takes place under peculiar circumstances and when the disorder is of extreme severity;" * as well as to show that our explanation of the transformation of gray into yellow tubercle, and the softening of tubercles with consequent destruction of pulmonary tissue by secondary inflammation is not rendered untenable by the observations of NIEMEYER.

* See volume before referred to, p. 217.

CHAPTER III.

TREATMENT OF CONSUMPTION.

Seeing that cod liver oil, whiskey, and other fashionable medicinal agents are far from being reliable in the treatment of this disease, a sense of obligation to the honor and integrity of our humane profession, and to the welfare of the suffering and dying victims of consumption, behooved me to the study and cultivation of this disease in quest of something curative, in addition to our elaborate category of palliative medicines. And I now take great pleasure in candidly stating that I feel confident of suggesting a great improvement upon even the most recent therapeutics, by recommending to the profession nitric and muriatic acids in the treatment of pulmonary phthisis.

In regard to the medical properties of these agents, the reader is referred to works on therapeutics. For the present I will recapitulate briefly some of the opinions of a few of the most eminent authorities. Nitric acid is tonic and antiseptic, having been successfully used in typhus and malarial fevers.

"Dr. ARNOLDI, of Montreal, proposed it as almost a specific remedy for *whooping cough*, and his recommenda-

tions have been sustained by Drs. GIBB, WITSELL, ACHER-
LY, MENELLY, NOBLE, and others. Under its use the violence of the paroxysms is said to be greatly mitigated, and
the duration of the disease abridged by more than one-half.
In *chronic bronchitis*, with exhaustion of the system, and
a frequent harrassing and paroxysmal cough, Dr. GLOVER
derived material advantage from the employment of this
agent. Five or six drops of nitric acid in a glass of
sweetened water, taken twice a day, has been highly recommended for the removal of *hoarseness* in singers." *

It has been highly eulogized for its efficacy in syphilis
and chronic affections of the liver, on the hypothesis that
its action was somewhat like that of mercury. And in the
treatment of fatty degeneration of the liver, previously
mentioned as being a frequent concomitant of phthisis, Dr.
C. J. B. WILLIAMS, of London, recommends "nitric and
nitro-muriatic acids upon the hypothesis of their being of
an opposite nature to fat, thus affording abundance of oxygen which may remove a part of the superfluous fat, at the
same time supplying azote, which may contribute to the
formation of a more highly animalized plasma."†

And I will add that this highly animalized plasma, for
whose production under such circumstances these acids
are unquestionably competent, is quite desirable in consumptive cases, for many reasons. The objection might

* "Stillé's Materia Medica, 3d Ed., Vol. 1, p. 255.
† Williams' Principles of Medicine, p. 375.

be urged upon a superficial examination of the subject, that simply because they are "of an opposite nature to fat," they would therefore be opposed in their action to cod liver oil and all such articles; indeed, counteracting their effects, rendering these agents antagonistic and incompatible. Not so, however. Be it remembered that the action of these acids in their attack upon fats in the liver is in cases in which the fats exist in excess—as "*specific deposits.*"

Moreover, this action is a peculiar and elective one—I will not say specific—on deposits in a specific organ, constituting one of the pointed features of the disease, and this attack upon these products may, of course, be made by an agent having this special action, and at the same time whose general effect is tonic and antiphosphatic.

CHAPMAN and RAYER speak in the most eulogistic manner of the internal use of nitric acid in the treatment of *impetigo* and scrofulous sores presenting a cancerous aspect, after all other forms of treatment had signally failed; supposing its virtues to depend upon its furnishing azote in a concentrated form, at the same time being an alterant, thus promoting the formation of the nutritive fluids.

And in the treatment of the degraded condition of the fibrine, before quoted from Dr. WILLIAMS, both when it depends upon ordinary causes, or "when it depends upon the presence of a febriferous or putrescent poison in the system," this eminent clinician recommends these two agents, in the first instance on this hypothesis: " Which, from their power in stopping passive hemorrhage, in augmenting the muscular substance and strength, and in causing the healing of phagedenic and flabby ulcers, seem to have some more direct means of promoting the formation of the plasma of the blood than by their mere operation on the digestive organs." And in the second instance he says: "Their beneficial operation is probably connected with their antiseptic as well as with their stimulating power." *

"As nitric acid dissolves both uric acid and the phosphates, it was supposed to be applicable in those cases of gravel in which the uric acid and phosphates are mixed." †

And in support of its antiphosphatic‡ virtues, such eminent authorities as GOLDING BIRD, BRODIE, and others may be cited.

* Williams' Principles of Medicine, p. 160.
† U. S. Disp., 11th Ed., p. 47.
‡ Prof. BARTHOLOW, while agreeing with Prof. J. H. BENNETT and other pathologists that the derangement of digestion incident to phthisical cases consists in part of excessive acidity, says that this condition prevents the oxydation of the phosphates, which "change" he considers necessary to prepare them for assimilation; and that in such cases the *mineral* acids are indicated, owing to their tonic and oxygenating properties.
The objection to the use of nitric acid in cases in which there is already acidity of the stomach—and such cases are quite common—is not well taken ; for I am fully persuaded that in these cases on account of the atonic condition of that organ, the food is allowed to remain in it more than the normal length of time, thus preventing digestion, and causing, as Prof. Chambers says, "chemical decomposition." Thus it is evident that the " excessive acidity" is but the direct result of *fermentation* of the food in the stomach: and this abnormal process these acids are happily calculated to counteract, both on chemical and therapeutical grounds.

In regard to the medical properties of muriatic acid, I would say that they are somewhat similar to those of nitric acid, it being tonic, antiseptic, antiphosphatic, cholagogue, etc. I use this agent merely as an adjuvant to nitric acid, on account of those properties just mentioned, adhering more tenaciously to nitric acid as being of greater utility on account of its highly reputed efficacy in "*whooping cough, chronic bronchitis*, and the *hoarseness* of singers," showing 'that it exerts a peculiar soothing influence on the irritable state of the lungs, probably in the same way that chlorate of potash thus acts on irritable conditions of the larynx, or through some such peculiar agency.

Again, the most approved diet for consumptives in modern practice has been beef-steak, mutton-chops, veal-cutlets, and other articles of the nitrogenous variety. "Nitrogenized foods," says Thomas, "are substances containing nitrogen, and supposed to be the only substances capable of being converted into blood, and of forming organic tissues."*

This being the case, it will readily be seen, that inasmuch as "*nitric acid is the source whence all the other compounds of nitrogen are obtained*,"† the introduction of that agent into the stomach during primary digestion will render the food more highly nitrogenous by reacting upon the contents of the stomach, forming nitrates.

* Thomas' Med. Dictionary, page 359.
† Silliman's Principles of Chemistry, 32d Ed., p. 203.

Bearing somewhat on this point, I here quote a paragraph from a very sensible paper on the "Digestive Assimilation of Medicine," by Dr. W. J. ELSTUN, of Indianapolis, Indiana:

"Medicinal substances are assimilated by the same selective or physiological affinity, through which each organ selects from the blood the particular food material required for its own support, nourishment, or vitality."*

From the foregoing statements it will be seen that both these agents, more especially the nitric acid, are appropriate remedies for the treatment of all stages of the disease; their combined properties being appropriate in all, but more especially in the first and second stages when the tubercular matter is being formed and deposited. And in the third stage, when excavation is taking place, it does not seem improbable that their antiseptic properties should, to a certain extent, antagonize the breaking down of tissue that accompanies and constitutes a part of the process of suppuration and softening of tubercles, in the same way that those properties of *carbolic* acid thus act when locally applied.

If we have been correct in our mental conceptions as to the abnormal accumulation of the phosphates in subjects possessing the tuberculous diathesis, either acquired, or the product of hereditary taint, superinduced, of course, by the influence of debilitating and other causes, there

* Western Journal of Medicine, October, 1869, p. 619.

3

can be no difficulty in seeing how the imperfect phosphatic elimination gathering increased force consummates tuberculous deposits with all their attendant consequences.

Holding these views as to the cause and nature of the disease under consideration, the appropriateness of the *mineral* acids, and especially the *nitric*, becomes manifest at a glance. And I am glad to be able to candidly state that my experience in practice has so fully sustained the truth of these preconceived theories, that I do not deem it proper to detain the reader with any extended argument upon the subject. If the very brief and imperfect manner in which my views are presented in this monograph, accompanied by cases reported, shall lead my medical brethren to the faithful and continued employment of these remedies, I am so confident as to the favorable results to be obtained, that I shall await their verdict, by which I shall be content to stand or fall.

When we consider carefully and intelligently the precise relation of this pathology to these therapeutics, the practicability of this theory and utility of these agents becomes quite apparent, as will be shown by a subsequent report of cases.

As to the employment of these remedies. Nitric acid I administer in doses of 30 to 40 drops (beginning with less if the stomach is much enfeebled or very irritable,) of the officinal dilute, in a small glass of water immediately after each meal, for the purpose of aiding digestion, and for other reasons already given. The quantity of muriatic acid which I administer is contained in 25 to 30 drops of tincture of chloride of iron, giving this agent for the two-fold purpose of both the acid and iron, having it taken sufficiently diluted half an hour before each meal, thereby getting its stimulating or appetizing influence.

Finally, while I claim for these two agents a great degree of superiority over even the most recent recognized therapeutics (considering alcoholic stimulants as being worse than useless, except in cases of extreme exhaustion,*) I would also state that it is not my intention thus to supersede cod-liver oil, suitable food, good hygiene, and other valuable and important measures, but that the medicines by me suggested are intended only as adjuvants to other appropriate measures at the discretion of the practitioner. Neither do I propose, by this method of treatment, to cure "the tuberculous diathesis" any more than colchicum and the alkalies would cure "the rheumatic diathesis."

In support of the views herein given, see following tabulated report of cases :

* See Chapter IV.

Case.	Age.	Sex.	Temperament.	Social Condition.	Occupation.	Nativity.
1st	33	Male.	Bilious.	Married.	Clerk.	German.
2d	16	"	Nervo-sanguine.	Single.	Wireweaver	"
3d	26	Female.	Bilious.	Widow.	Teacher.	United States.
4th	17	Male.	Phlegmatic.	Single.	Apprentice at tailoring.	German.
5th	22	Female.	"	"	Saleswoman	United States.
6th	"	Male.	Nervo-sanguine.	"	Clerk.	England.
7th	27	Female.	Nervous.	Married.	Housework.	German.
8th	23	"	Nervo-sanguine.	Single.	Prostitute.	United States.
9th	14	"	Bilious.	"	Nurse.	Colored.
10th	18	"	Nervous.	"	Housework.	United States.
11th	32	"	Bilious.	Married.	"	"
12th	28	Male.	Nervous.	"	Laborer.	German.
13th	45	"	Bilious.	"	"	"

PHYSICAL CONDITION.	Length of time under treatment.	Result.
Dullness on percussion, rude inspiration, prolonged expiration, bronchial breathing, and broncophony over the upper two-thirds of superior lobe of left lung.	3 months.	Recovery.
Cracked-pot resonance, with cavernous respiration and pectoriloquy over the entire sup. ¼ of right lung. Also, dullness on percussion, rude inspiration, prolonged and jerking expiration, with occasional moist crackling at apex of left lung.	13 "	Recovery.
Slight dullness on percussion, rude and tremulous inspiration, and dry crackling on forced inspiration, with prolonged expiration at apex of left lung.	3 "	Recovered.
Broncophony and mucous rale approaching cavernous, with dullness on percussion over the sup. ⅔ of upper lobe of right lung. Also, friction rales and slight rudeness, and prolongation of the respiratory murmur, with slight dullness under left clavicle.	8 "	"
Decided dullness on percussion, with dry crackling and rude inspiration, while the expiratory effort was much prolonged over the upper part of the left chest. Also, sonorous and sibilant rales over both lungs.	6 "	"
Great dullness, with local depression, rude inspiration, and prolonged expiration at apex of right lung. The same, but less marked, on left side.	6¾ "	"
Dullness over the upper fourth of left lung, with rude inspiration, prolonged expiration, bronchial breathing, and bronchophony. Slight dullness, with rudeness and prolongation of respiratory sounds at right apex.	6 "	"
Considerable depression and dullness, with humid crackling, bronchial breathing, and bronchophony under right clavicle. Also, some evidence of deposit at other apex.	7½ "	"
Amphoric resonance, with cavernous respiration and pectoriloquy in sup. lobe of right lung. Dullness over entire left lung, mucous rale and ægophony over its sup. lobe.	2 "	Favorable.
. . . .	13 days.	Died.
Infiltrated tubercle diffused throughout the entire upper lobe of left lung. Cavernous respiration and pectoriloquy at apex of right lung.	7 months.	Favorable.
. . . .	6 weeks.	Died.
Considerable tubercular deposit at apex of both lungs.	5 months.	"

Case.	Age.	Sex.	Temperament.	Social Con-dition.	Occupation.	Nativity.
14th	44	Male.	Bilious.	Married.	Tinner.	United States.
15th	19	"	"	Single.	Laborer.	German.
16th	51	"	Nervo-sanguine.	Married.	"	United States.
17th	30	Female.	Bilious.	"	Domestic.	"
18th	23	Male.	"	"	Farmer.	"
19th	30	"	"	"	Mis'laneous	"
20th	43	"	Nervo-sanguine.	"	Book-keep'r	Scotland.
21st	26	"	Sanguine.	"	....	German.
22d	33	"	Bilious.	Single.	Clerk.	Scotland.
23d	49	Female.	Nervous.	Widow.	Domestic.	Irish.
24th	28	Male.	Bilious.	Married.	Merchant.	German.

PHYSICAL CONDITION.	Length of time under treatment.	Result.
Considerable flattening of thoracic wall, with dullness and other signs of tubercular deposit at apex of right lung. Same, but less marked, on left side.	4 months.	Recovered.
A cavity of considerable size, accompanied with the most unmistakable cracked-pot sound that I have ever met with, in the upper lobe of right lung. Also, dullness on percussion, rude inspiration, and prolonged expiration at apex of left lung.	6 "	Recovery.
Marked depression of thoracic wall antero-laterally, with profound dullness on percussion, bronchial breathing and broncophony over the entire space above the nipple on the right side. Exaggerated breathing on left side.	7 "	Favorable.
Dullness on percussion, rude inspiration and prolonged expiration at apices of both lungs. Dry crackling was also noticed upon forced inspiration at apex of the left lung.	7 "	"
Marked dullness on percussion, with bronchial breathing and broncophony over the superior half of the upper lobe of the left lung. Also, slight rudeness and prolongation of respiratory sounds at apex of right lung.	4⅔ "	".
Well marked tubercular deposit in the upper lobe of right lung. Slight deposit at apex of left lung.	4 "	".
Sibilant and sonorous rales, with slight dullness on percussion, and some rudeness and prolongation of respiratory sounds at apices of both lungs.	4 "	"
Marked dullness on percussion, bronchial breathing and broncophony over superior two-thirds of the upper lobe of left lung. Puerile respiration on right side.	2 "	Improved.
Cavernous respiration and pectoriloquy in superior lobe of right lung. Also, slight dullness on percussion, with harshness of respiratory murmur at apex of left lung.	4 "	Improving.
Dullness on percussion, bronchial breathing and broncophony in superior lobe of left lung. Circumscribed pectoriloquy in upper lobe of right lung.	3 "	"
Cavernous respiration and pectoriloquy in upper lobe of left lung. Dullness on percussion, rude inspiration, prolonged expiration, with dry crackling on forced inspiration at apex of right lung.	3 "	"

As stated in another part of this chapter, these cases were treated with nitric and muriatic acids, aided by various auxiliaries as counter-irritants, narcotics, expectorants, cod-liver oil where it was tolerated, etc.. using very little alcohol, however.

I may briefly mention, by way of comment upon *Case 1st*, that THOMPSON's *line* on the gums was noticed to have disappeared within a month from the time at which the treatment was commenced. Patient had no cough (except during the occurrence of *partial* pleuritic attacks) to indicate the presence of inflammatory action, therefore my diagnosis was tuberculosis of the gray variety; and the total disappearance of percussion dullness and abnormal respiratory sounds was in my estimation, "proof positive" of the antiphosphatic virtues of the treatment. This patient, like all the others, was very much emaciated.

Case 2d was emaciated to the most profound degree. Gained ten pounds more than his original weight within the first six months of medication, and pursued his occupation during the day and attended night school in the evening throughout the winter. When I last saw him a casual examination indicated some evidence of pulmonary lesion, but being able to work, he concluded to discontinue medication; he had improved in his physical as well as general condition.

Case 3d had been in bad health during three years preceding, at which time she had a miscarriage with great loss of blood. Several months after discharging her, I received a letter from her stating that her health was then "quite as good as ever."

Case 4th, being a scrofulous subject, took *syr. ferri iodidi* instead of *tr. ferri chloridi.* At time of dismission, although his general health was good, there was still evidence of lesion in right lung.

Case 5th had been able to pursue her occupation *without fatigue* six weeks prior to dismission, while the catamenia had for three months been perfectly natural.

Case 6th was a perfect success, except a slight flatness under right clavicle.

Cases 7th and 8th made good recoveries.

Case 9th improved rapidly while under my treatment, but in two months, owing to her removal to a distant part of the country, she passed from my further observation.

Case 10th was a young lady aged 18, referred to the writer by Prof. H. E. FOOTE. This case was diagnosticated both by the Professor and myself as one of advanced consumption, there being so much intra-thoracic tenderness, however, that we were unable to make any satisfactory physical examination, and therefore cannot report the physical condition of the lungs. This patient evinced a slow, but constant improvement, notwithstanding she had been confined to her bed for four weeks previous, and was so anæmic that any amount of friction applied to the surface would not redden it. On the eleventh day of treatment, in sponging the skin, it was noticed to react to the friction thereby applied. The next day she was able to sit up in bed, and on the following day I gave her permission to sit up in an arm-chair properly prepared with blankets, etc., during an interval of half an hour in both forenoon and afternoon. Feeling remarkably well, (under the circum- stances) she sat up much longer than I had directed, "caught cold," the cough was fearfully aggravated, and at 9 P. M. died from apnœa.

" *Case* 11*th*, notwithstanding her unfavorable sanitary surroundings, is the most satisfactory case of any kind that I have ever treated. She occasionally expectorates cretaceous tubercles, which occasioned great inconvenience, suffocation, etc., prior to my attendance; but now when they are expectorated, it is done with the utmost facility. This, I think, is due to the antiphosphatic virtues of the treatment. For further comment on this point, see para- graph on '*modus operandi*' at close of these remarks."

The remarks contained in the above paragraph were made on the case when it was published in the *Phila- delphia Medical and Surgical Reporter* and Cincinnati *Lancet and Observer* a year ago. Dr. WM. CARSON ex- amined the case and confirmed our statement in a report to the Academy of Medicine. Soon after our report to the Academy of Medicine, however, the extreme meagre- ness of the patient's resources compelled her to discon- tinue the treatment, as she was unable even to purchase medicine or obtain appropriate food. She had, however, a compensating consolation in her poverty that she was tired of medication and able to work. She then began work for the performance of which her physical capacity was inadequate, as two, three or more days washing per week, which, as might reasonably be expected, (especially as she had not been *entirely* cured) caused a relapse of the disease from which she died, after having again been under treatment from September to May. Although as just stated, the case finally terminated fatally, nevertheless we feel warranted in reporting it "favorable" in the table, for the result of no case could be more favorable to or vindicative of the treatment than this while the patient was still within the reach of medicine. I will also state that during the last eight months of treatment the patient resided in a dark, damp, and oftentimes wet basement, in close proximity with the river, by which it is sometimes overflowed, and although the sanitary surroundings of her residence were before reported as being unfavorable when she resided in the attic of a large tenement house, yet it cannot be doubted that they were very much worse when she took up her abode in the basement.

Case 12*th* was so low that I was unable to make any satisfactory physical examination. He had been unable to eat or sleep satisfactorily for three months previous to my attendance, and neither appetite nor rest could be obtained, the latter by narcotics, of which all were tried in maximum doses, but without avail; he gradually failed and died at the end of the sixth week of medication.

Case 13*th* was a man broken down by debauchery, and had obstinate dyspepsia. At time of publication a year ago he was marked "stationary." Since that time, while "on a spree," he was subjected to exposure, after which followed a retrogressive action, terminating in death.

Case 14*th* was also broken down by debauchery, but nevertheless the results of treatment were of the most satisfactory character. In seven weeks from beginning the treatment he went to work, and during the first week that he was working he gained two-and-a-half pounds, notwithstanding his having previously been given up by a leading homœopathic physician, and subsequently by an eminent medical professor of Cincinnati.

Case 15*th* applied to me for treatment while visiting some friends in the country in the early part of July, 1870. He was as might be supposed, very much emaciated, and the cracked-pot sound referred to in the table was so marked as to be noticed even by unprofessional bystanders when I directed their attention to it.

I ordered tincture of the chloride of iron, one ounce, with sulphate of quinia half a drachm, 20 to 30 drops of the mixture to be taken in a small glass of water half an hour before each meal. Also 30 to 40 drops of dilute nitric acid in the same quantity of water after each meal, and when his digestion should have sufficiently improved, a tablespoonful of cod liver oil three-quarters of an hour after having taken the acid. As an expectorant, I prescribed a mixture composed of equal quantities of syrup of lactucarium and syrup of prunus virginiana, a tea to a dessertspoonful of which was to be taken when required to relieve cough.

He promised to keep me informed by mail as to the progress of his case, but as I did not hear from him, I concluded that he must have either decided not to take the medicine or had died. In the latter part of January, 1871, however, while again visiting in the same vicinity, I was told that soon after my visit in July he left that part of the country for the purpose of residing with his relatives in one of the eastern States, and that he had not been heard from until a few days before, while a steamboat was landed for a few moments in the vicinity of his old home, when he presented himself on the guard of the boat near which two of his old associates were standing on the landing, who, as he had improved so much, would not have known him had he not introduced himself to them. In the table his case is reported as one of recovery, and although we are not acquainted with the present condition of his lungs, we feel warranted, from what he told the two gentlemen in their brief interview concerning his general condition, in reporting the case as one of recovery.

Case 16*th* presented a more marked retraction antero-laterally of the entire thoracic wall above the right nipple than I have ever witnessed in any other case. He had

been quite unwell for several years, having been delicate
from childhood, and had been treated by quite a number of
leading physicians of all schools, none of whom ever did
him any good except to palliate the severity of his ailments.
The treatment of this case did not vary essentially from
that of the one preceding, except that compound tincture
of gentian was frequently alternated with the iron and
quinine solution, and tincture of iodine or tartar emetic
ointment were occasionally employed to remedy the intra-
thoracic tenderness, which at times, especially in the beginning, was very severe. At the end of seven months he
discontinued medication, feeling tolerably well, and having
improved very much not only as regarded his general condition but the physical condition of his affected lung also.
Upon a physical examination of his chest recently (four
months since he was under treatment) I found the percussion dullness very much diminished and the infra-clavi-
cular retraction less marked, while his general health is
good, permitting him to do a full day's work without any
particular fatigue.

Case 17*th* was a woman who would not take her medicine regularly, but when she did follow directions for a
while, the result was always of the most flattering character—there being improvement in her appearance and
general condition, and diminution in lassitude, anorexia,
and severity of cough. Owing, in my judgment, to the
fact that this patient could not be induced to take her

medicine perseveringly, no decided advantage over her disease has been gained, there still being evidence of decided pulmonary trouble. Nevertheless, its progress has manifestly been retarded, and the patient's life thus prolonged. I regret exceedingly that the full benefits of the treatment have not been secured, as I am very sanguine they would have been complete. Hence the case is marked "favorable" in the table ; for when my directions were strictly obeyed, the results of no case could be more in favor of the treatment.

Case 18*th* was several weeks under observation before there was the slightest evidence of improvement. The dorsum of his tongue was covered with a thin whitish fur so frequently observed in subjects of the disease. I was, therefore, led to prescribe three grain doses of blue mass every second or third night at bed time, followed the next morning with a saline cathartic, administering the anti-tuberculous remedies in the mean time. At length, the tongue cleaned off, breathing became easier, and there was marked general improvement of all his symptoms continuing most satisfactorily for about four months, at which time a most thorough physical examination was made. The rudeness and prolongation of respiratory sounds manifested by the right lung at previous examinations had now disappeared, and the field of percussion dullness presented by his left lung was diminished. So I regarded his convalescence as thoroughly established. He now passed from

under my observation, going into the interior of a neighboring State where I have not been able to get his address
and cannot, therefore, state his present condition.

Case 19th was a laborer employed in work of a miscel-
laneous character, frequently suffering undue fatigue and
exposure, which obviously counteracted to some extent the
benefit of treatment. A few weeks after he came under
my charge, he was seized with a most violent hæmoptysis,
for the relief of which the remedies usually recommended
were employed without avail; the hemorrhage recurring
from time to time threatening the most serious consequences. At this juncture of the case I sought the advice
of Prof. WM. H. MUSSEY, at whose suggestion the following
formula was administered:

R. Persulphate of iron, - - - ∋j.
 Alum, - - - - - ∋ij.
 Powdered gum acacia, - - ∋j.
 White sugar, - - - - ∋ij.
Mix and triturate thoroughly. Divide into twenty pow-
ders, one of which was to be administered at intervals
of from thirty to sixty minutes, according to the seve-
rity of the hemorrhage.

The result was most salutary. In similar cases a little
opium or laudanum may be added to the above with advantage. Notwithstanding the unfavorable symptoms here
detailed, this patient after four months' treatment according to my general plan was so far recovered as to enable
him to enter upon the occupation of a huckster, the duties

of which he has been able to perform with but little interruption to the present time. From a letter to one of his friends in the vicinity a short time since (six months after dismission) I learned that his condition is constantly improving.

Case 20*th* was a case of tuberculosis, complicated with bronchitis. The treatment was in every respect a perfect success.

Case 21*st* was a man completely broken down by debauchery; his drinking was almost without limit, and was indulged in at night as well as day. I had him under treatment two months, inducing him to reduce his drinks to three small glasses of brandy per day, one immediately after each dose of cod liver oil—the nitric acid administered as usual. During the whole time improvement was most marked. He could, however, no longer be held to habits of temperance, but has alternated between rioting and dissipation, neglecting his medicine, and attempts to abstain from drinking and use the treatment ordered up to the present time; dissipation having almost constant supremacy. Although, as before stated, he improved satisfactorily while under treatment, and temperate habits were observed, we can, as might be expected under the circumstances, claim but little if any *permanent* advantage from the treatment.

Case 22*d* has been a subject of the disease for over three years. He had tried every form of treatment usually

4

practiced, with no other than palliative results. As the
patient resides in Chicago, and on account of his extensive
engagements cannot take time to come and see me per-
sonally, I have to rely for information concerning the progress of his case upon an epistolary correspondence. I
heard from him a few days ago, when he was still improving in a very satisfactory manner. I cannot, however, on
account of the facts just mentioned, give the present physical condition of his lungs.

   Case 23*d* is an elderly lady, of very limited means, and
not, therefore, able to procure all the dietetic and hygienic
adjuvants to the medical treatment that would be desirable. She has, however, notwithstanding the fact that
she was scarcely able to walk across her room when she
first consulted me, constantly improved in every particular. The " circumscribed pectoriloquy " mentioned
in the table seems to be limited to a very small space.
With the stethoscope in a certain position, it can be
quite distinctly heard ; but if the instrument be moved as
much as the width of the trumpet-shaped end of an ordinary stethoscope, the sound ceases to be audible, on account,
as I believe, of the cavity being small, and most distinctly
heard when it is situated immediately under the centre
of the stethoscope.

   Case 24*th.* This man had labored under the disease for
over two years. Besides emaciation, the physical signs
unmistakably testified to the advancement of the malady

toward a fatal termination. He suffered greatly from indigestion, for which I prescribed subnitrate of bismuth
(8 or 9 grains), with BOUDAULT's pepsin (6 or 7 grains),
immediately after eating (it may be taken *just before* eat-
ing), followed with thirty to forty drops of dilute nitric
acid, taken through a glass or cane tube, after having
diluted it in a small glass of water, about forty minutes
after administering the bismuth and pepsin. He was also
allowed tincture of iron and quinine, as in some of the foregoing cases. He was under observation for a period of
nine weeks, during which time there was decided improvement in all the physical signs, and a corresponding gain in
strength and weight. He then passed from my observation, continuing the treatment on his own responsibility.
At last accounts (by mail) he was still improving, "having
gained four (4) pounds in weight" during an interval of
eight days. I feel warranted, at least, in reporting this
case as "favorable."

As a gentleman in the "Academy of Medicine," when
our report was presented, was unable to understand that
the lungs when once invaded could ever be freed from
tubercular deposit, it may be well to say a few words in
regard to the *modus operandi* of this treatment as regards
the removal of tubercular deposit.

Dr. LAWSON, in regard to this matter, makes the two
following propositions : " *To promote the elimination of
tuberculous matter ;*" " *To promote the absorption of tuber-*

cles."* For this purpose he recommends various alterants, as iodine, bromine, alkalies, mercurials, sarsaparilla, etc. And for the removal of inflammatory products (for it will be remembered that according to either NIEMEYER's or my own theory the caseous matter of crude tubercles is the result of inflammation), Dr. C. J. B. WILLIAMS recommends these agents and goes on to state that he " can affirm from much experience in its use that *nitric acid* is the best medicine " he knows of for this purpose, supposing its action in part to be by "further oxygenating them."† On this point, also see some of the notes at the bottom of previous pages.

* Lawson's Treatise on Consumption, pp. 448 and 456.
† Williams' Principles of Medicine, p. 346.

CHAPTER IV.

ALCOHOL IN CONSUMPTION.

In a previous chapter we alluded to "alcoholic stimulants as being worse than useless except in cases of extreme
exhaustion." We will now give our reasons for that opinion. In the chapter above referred to, we showed that as
the plasma of the blood "is the basis of the constructive
and reparative process," the principal thing to be done in
the treatment of that disease is to promote the formation
of the fibrin; a process which under the circumstances is
very imperfectly performed, and, as will hereafter be seen,
is rendered still more so by the influence of alcoholic
liquors. What are some of the

EFFECTS OF ALCOHOLIC LIQUORS

and the changes produced by them in the tissues and
fluids of the body? "The most important physical change,"
says Dr. CARPENTER ("by contact) is that of corrugation;
due to the difference in facility with which alcohol and
water respectively pass through animal membranes." "The
corrugating effect is usually increased by the coagulating

influence exerted on whatever soluble albumen may be contained in the tissues, and is proportioned in their degree to the state of concentration of the alcohol; but some such physical change must always take place in the walls of the stomach whenever alcoholic fluids are introduced into it, and in the soft tissues of the body at large, whenever alcohol has found its way into the current of the circulation*"

That alcohol finds "its way into the current of the circulation," and in larger quantity than is generally supposed, can admit of no doubt, since we have before us the following ocular demonstration: "in so far as we are acquainted with the powers of the stomach, we have no evidence that it is capable of digesting or decomposing alcohol. Dr. BEAUMONT, in his experiments with St. Martin, observed that neither alcohol nor fermented liquors, nor other *fluids*, not holding aliment in solution, are changed by the gastric juice, but very soon after being received, pass out of the stomach either through the pylorus or by absorption— . . . it is to be inferred that no healthy animal process whatever can accomplish its dissolution.

* Alcohol, like heat, acids, etc., it is well known, coagulates albumen whenever they are brought in contact; so in the culinary preparation of food as well as in the process of digesting it, the albumen becomes coagulated;—in the former instance by the application of heat, in the latter by the action of the acids of the stomach. But later in the process of digestion, we find that pepsin, the active principle of the gastric juice, renders the already coagulated albumen soluble by converting it into albuminose. "The coagulating influence," however, referred to in the above paragraph, cannot be remedied by pepsin, as it is exerted upon *the albumen of the blood* after the "alcohol has found its way into the current of the circulation." Carpenter's Prize Essay on Alcoholic Liquors, pp. 25, 26.

In the stomach it is alcohol, in the *lungs* it is alcohol, in the brain it is alcohol."*

The experiments of RUDOLPH MASING, since repeated and confirmed by MM. LALLEMAND, PERRIN, and DUROY, have taught us that alcohol passes through the body unaltered in its chemical constitution; and Prof. N. S. DAVIS,† of Chicago, says that this position is now acknowledged to be correct by all classes of observers; and additional support is afforded to these positions by the researches of Dr. PERCY, who found that the tissues remote from the stomach became impregnated with alcohol when it passed into the current of the circulation.‡

GRAVES cites a case where a clear fluid which had the taste and smell of alcohol was found in the ventricles of the brain, and which ignited on being brought near a burning body.§

Coincident with this, a striking example of the apparent presence of alcohol in the blood is mentioned by Dr. MUS-SEY. A medical friend of his bled a man who had been drinking freely for three or four days. The halitus of the blood burned for thirty seconds, with a blue flame, on the application of a lighted taper.‖

Finding "its way into the current of the circulation,"

---

* " Mussey's Prize Essay on Ardent Spirits," p. 27.
† *Chicago Medical Examiner*, March, 1871, p. 130.
‡ See Experimental Inquiry Concerning the Presence of Alcohol in the Ventricles of the Brain, p. 29.
§ Studies, Etc. p. 315.
‖ Trans. Amer. Med. Assoc. VIII, 575.

what changes are produced in the quality, especially of the plastic elements of the blood? "Among the most important of the chemical changes which alcohol has the power of effecting, is the coagulation of soluble albumen : and although it will rarely, if ever, be introduced into the mass of the blood, or into the serous fluid of the tissues, by any ordinary alcoholic potations, in a sufficiently concentrated state to effect this, yet we should anticipate that its presence, even in a very dilute form, must affect the chemical relations of albumen, and can scarcely do otherwise than retard that peculiar transformation by which it is converted into the more vitalized substance, Fibrine." *" No considerable changes* [italics ours] *of a physical or chemical nature can take place in any of the animal tissues, without disordering their vital properties also;* and we now have to inquire into the mode in which these properties are affected by the contact of alcoholic liquors. In the first place, it would appear that the solidifiability of the fibrine, which is its special vital endowment, is impaired by the introduction of alcohol into the fluid which contains it; for when an animal is killed by the injection of alcohol into the blood-vessels, the blood often remains fluid after death, or coagulates* but imperfectly. Now, as it is probable that nearly all the organized tissues are developed at the expense of

---

* "When a draught of alcoholic liquor proves fatal, the blood in the heart, the large vessels, and the lungs, is entirely fluid; so effectual is this poison in preventing the last natural act of vitality in the blood, its coagulation." (Mussey's Prize Essay on Ardent Spirits, p. 23.)

the fibrine, it is obvious that anything which impairs its organizability must have an injurious influence upon the general nutritive operations."*

" There are some peculiar effects of Alcohol upon the blood, besides its influence on the coagulability of the fibrine, of which it is proper that special mention should be made.   When alcohol is mingled with fresh arterial blood, it darkens its color, so as to give it more or less of a venous aspect.   And when this admixture is made under the microscope, it is observed that the red corpuscles shrink, and that a considerable part of their contents becomes mingled with the liquor sanguinis.   Now, although the peculiar functions of the red corpuscles have not yet been precisely determined by physiologists, there is no doubt whatever that they are among the most important constituents of the blood; and there is strong reason to believe that they are subservient on the one hand to the respiratory function, and on the other, either directly or indirectly, to the elaboration† of the *plasma* or organizable material of the blood.   It is highly improbable, then, that any considerable effect can be produced upon them, without seriously impairing the processes of aeration and nutri-

* Carpenter's Prize Essay on Alcoholic Liquors, pp. 26 and 27.
† Owing to the fact that they carry oxygen in arterial blood, and the plasma being a deutoxide of proteine, it seems "that they are subservient to the elaboration of the plasma" by virtue of their oxygen.   And the correctness of this hypothesis is proven by the demonstrative fact that a substance identical with fibrine in every respect may be prepared by chemical manipulation in which oxygen is made to act upon albumen.

tion; both of which are prejudicially influenced in other ways, by the presence of alcohol in the blood."*

In the preceding paragraph the effects of alcohol on fresh drawn arterial blood as revealed by "the microscope" are given : "*the admixture of alcohol with the blood has a tendency* [italics ours] *to give a venous character even to that of the arteries;* and when this tendency is augmented by imperfect respiration [*as is the case* in the disease under consideration], *the blood will become more and more venous.*" † And to show the completeness of "this tendency," it is worthy of remark that alcohol introduced into the system of a cock or turkey, will cause the comb and wattles of the birds to lose their bright crimson or scarlet hue, and become purple and dusky. (And for additional authority on this point, see Stillé's Materia Medica, Third Edition, Vol. 1, p. 629; Annuaire de Thérap., 1862, p. 212; and Liebig's Animal Chemistry, Philadelphia Edition, p. 71.)

This venous condition of arterial blood within the body is doubtless produced, as CARPENTER has explained, through the wonderful facility with which alcohol is oxydized; since it will withdraw the oxygen from other substances which are waiting to be eliminated by the combustive process, besides the antiseptic influence which it exerts on such substances, preventing or retarding chemical

---

* Carpenter's Prize Essay on Alcoholic Liquors, p. 29.
† Ibid. p. 36.

changes in them, the accumulation of which will deterio-
rate the character of the fluid.   That such is the case is
shown by the experiments of BOUCHARDAT, who found that
when alcohol is introduced into the system (perhaps in
moderate, or even in larger quantities), the blood in the
arteries presents the aspect of venous blood, showing with
certainty that it has been prevented from undergoing the
proper oxygenating process.   And the experiments of Dr.
PROUT afford additional support to this conclusion; for, no
sooner had the effects of the alcohol passed off, than he observed that the quantity of carbonic acid exhaled arose
much above the normal standard—thus giving, it would
seem, unequivocal evidence of the previous abnormal retention of carbonaceous matter in the system.

One of the principal reasons given for employing alcoholic liquors in the treatment of consumption is that " it

RETARDS THE RETROGRADE METAMORPHOSIS OF TISSUE,

and therefore checks destructive metamorphosis, and gives
time to build up with beef and iron."   The fallacy of this
notion becomes quite apparent when we consider the well-
established fact that while it retards *de*structive, it also has
the same effect on *con*structive metamorphosis.   And Prof.
CHAMBERS, of London, in support of this view cites the
well-known fact that " alcohol is given to puppies to keep

them small dogs,* and it is stated that dwarf-like jockeys have been produced by the same treatment. We have thus a warning of what the effect of the agent is."† BIG-LAND, in his Natural History, informs us that "the elephants exhibited in Europe are commonly of a diminutive size;" and that they are exceedingly fond of spirituous liquors. One of them, he says, was habituated to the daily consumption of twelve [12] pints of wine; and another at the Exeter 'Change in 1803, "was so excessively fond of beer that he has been known to drink upwards of fifty [50] quarts in a day, given by his numerous visitors." We also notice that the growth of boys is not unfrequently stunted by their falling victims to "intemperate" habits.

As alcohol increases venosity, and at the same time disorganizes the red corpuscles, of course it cannot, by interfering with "oxydation" (to which we have elsewhere referred), do otherwise than prevent the normal formation of the fibrine; and it is by the influence thus exerted, as well as by that described in a succeeding part of this chapter, on

---

* Dr. H. W. Fowler, of this city, informs me of the following case: A small terrier slut was in labor three days with terrible pains, and died without delivery. A post-mortem examination revealed good development, there being no deformity whatever. The pups, however, of which there were three, were found to be preternaturally large, causing the failure of delivery. The owner of the bitch had been careful that she should be copulated by a small dog. Upon inquiry, however, he found that the owner of the dog employed had kept him stunted in growth by alcoholic potations, so that the smallness of his size was not due to his breed, and his progeny were measured by his stock and not by his size.

† Chambers on the Renewal of Life, p. 51.

the nervous system, that we explain its *modus operandi* as a retarder of *con*structive metamorphosis of tissue.

A prominent feature in our discussion so far, drawing from the opinions of the most eminent authorities, has been to show that both by its peculiar and destructive action upon the albumen and red corpuscles, and its tendency to increase venosity of the blood, alcohol prevents or retards the normal formation of the blood plasma.   Let us consider briefly some of the

EFFECTS OF DEFICIENT PLASTICITY OF THE BLOOD.

One complication very much to be dreaded in the management of this disease is the occurrence of pulmonary hemorrhage.   The statement of Dr. CARPENTER that "certain forms of hemorrhage are obviously dependent in part on insufficient plasticity," affords a partial explanation of this form of hemorrhage.

Next note some of its baneful effects on nutrition.   Under the head of " Diminished Power of Sustaining Injuries by Disease or Accident," Dr. CARPENTER says: " The classes of men among whom there is an appearance of remarkable bodily vigor, notwithstanding habitual excess in the use of alcoholic liquors, are those who are continually undergoing great muscular exertion, and who not only drink largely, but eat heartily.   Of this class the London Coal-heavers, Ballasters, and Brewers' Draymen are remarkable examples. Many of them drink from two to three gallons of porter daily, and even spirits besides. They are, for the most part, large, gross, unwieldy men, and are capable of great bodily exertion, so long, at least, as their labor is carried on in the *open air*. But it does not hence follow that they are in a condition of real vigor; for the constitutions of such men break down before they are far advanced in years, even if they do not earlier fall victims (as a large proportion of them do) to the results of disease or injury which were at first apparently of the most trifling character. It is well known . . . that when such men suffer from inflammatory attacks, or local injuries, these are peculiarly disposed to run on to a fatal termination, in consequence, it is evident, of the deficient plasticity of the blood. . . . . The want of plasticity of the blood gives the inflammatory processes an *asthenic* instead of a *sthenic* character; there is no limitation by plastic effusion, but they spread far and wide through the tissues. . . . Thus we see that in such men the slightest scratch or bruise will not unfrequently give rise to a fatal attack of erysipelas; and that internal organs affected with inflammation rapidly become infiltrated with pus, or pass into a gangrenous state."*

So, in our opinion, the lungs "affected with inflammation" by the presence of tubercle or vicissitudes of temperature, with deficient plasticity of the blood (although a sufficient quantity of food *may* have been eaten, as in the

---

* Carpenter's Prize Essay on Alcoholic Liquors, pp. 65 and 66.

cases just cited, but not properly digested and elaborated, as the reader will understand), and this pathological condition being still further aggravated by the introduction of alcohol into the blood, it would seem clear that their tendency "to become infiltrated with pus or pass into a gangrenous state" will thereby be increased. So much for alcohol producing deficient plasticity, which must necessarily occasion malnutrition of the body.

We will now consider the

EFFECTS OF ALCOHOL ON THE NUTRITION OF THE NERVOUS SYSTEM.

"Its special power of exciting the *nervous centres* to augmented activity, can only be accounted for by the idea of some special relation between alcohol and nervous matter.* And this idea is fully borne out by the fact that Dr. PERCY found alcohol to exist in the substance of the brains of dogs poisoned by it, in considerably greater proportion than in an equivalent quantity of blood. This fact is one of fundamental importance, as showing us how directly and immediately the whole nutrition and vital activity of the nervous system must be affected by the presence of alcohol in the blood—the alcohol being thus speedily

---

* "It may be almost positively affirmed, that notwithstanding the chemical relation which alcohol bears to nervous matter, it cannot serve, either in its original condition, or under any other guise, as a *pabulum* for the generation of nervous tissue." Carpenter's Prize Essay on Alcoholic Liquors, p. 83.

drawn out of the circulating current by the nervous matter, and incorporated with its substance in such a manner
as even to change, when in sufficient amount, its physical
as well as its chemical properties. It is important, also,
to observe that this affinity is obviously such as will occasion the continual presence of alcohol in the blood, even
in very minute proportion, to modify the nutrition of the
nervous substance more than that of any other tissue; for
the alcohol will *seek out*, as it were, the nervous matter,
and will fasten upon it,—just as we see that other poisons,
whose *results* become more obvious to our senses, (although
the poisons themselves may exist in such minute amount
as not to be detectible by the most refined analysis,) will
localize themselves in particular organs, or even in particular spots of the same organ."*

The same author, in speaking of delirium tremens, says,
" that the disease is as much dependent upon the *disordered
state of nutrition*, more particularly that of the nervous
substance, as before shown, consequent upon the habitual
presence of alcohol in the blood, as it is upon the positive
exhaustion of nervous power consequent upon the violence
of the excitement, which is the more immediate effect of
the stimulus."   On the same page, in speaking of insanity,
" *at least a quarter* of the whole number of cases" of which,
he says, may be assigned to the habitual employment of
alcoholic liquors, and that "their action on the system is

* Carpenter's Prize Essay on Alcoholic Liquors, pp. 35 and 36.

that of slowly and imperceptibly modifying its *nutritive* operations, so as gradually to alter the chemical, physical, and, thereby, the vital properties of the fabric, and thus to prepare it for being acted upon by causes which, in the healthy condition, produce no influence."* " If the nerves . . . be inadequately nourished, it is impossible that their normal power can be developed, except under the influence of stimulants, and then only for a short time."†

On this point Prof. CHAMBERS says: " We can hardly hesitate to call alcohol an arrester of nerve-life, and consequently a controller of nervous action on the rest of the frame."‡   And Dr. EDWARD SMITH, an eminent authority on this subject, after a series of carefully conducted experiments, says : " Temperate men, after taking brandy with a fasting stomach, always have lessened consciousness, lessened sensibility to sound, to light, and to touch, and there is a peculiar sensation of stiffness in the lips and cheeks ;" and it is exceedingly common for drinking men to determine how much they are under the influence of alcoholic drinks by the degree of numbness they experience in passing the fingers over their cheeks.   The author, who is to no extent whatever habitually addicted to ardent spirits, would also state that these effects, especially the last, have been produced in his own person by a single glass of lager-beer.

* Carpenter's Prize Essay on Alcoholic Liquors, p. 42.
† Ibid. p. 82.
‡ Chambers on Renewal of Life. Second American ed., p. 600.

It is also worthy of mention here, inasmuch as it corroborates the foregoing statements, especially the one last quoted from Prof. CHAMBERS, that recently at the sitting of the Paris Academy of Medicine, M. GALEZOWSKI pointed out the frequency of his observation of impaired vision (amblyopia) from " chronic," not excessive, use of alcoholic drinks.

Having seen that alcohol interferes with its nutrition, and consequently diminishes its functional power, let us consider briefly the importance of the

INFLUENCE OF THE NERVOUS SYSTEM

on the general nutrition of the body.

The most palpable examples of defective nutrition from want of nervous energy are observed in cases of paralyzed limbs. And while deficient exercise of the parts undoubtedly accounts in part for their atrophied condition, yet there are good reasons for believing that the inadequate excitation from the injured nerves is the chief cause of atrophy in such cases. Limited space will not admit of our entering into an extensive discussion of this subject, but we will cite a few cases in point that will not be without weight. Lesions of the spinal cord are sometimes followed by mortification of portions of the paralyzed parts ; and this may take place very quickly, as in a case by Sir B. BRODIE,[*]

* Brodie's Lectures on Pathology and Surgery. Longmans, 1846, p. 309.

in which the ankle sloughed within twenty-four hours after an injury of the spine. A similar case is recorded by Mr. CURLING in the twentieth volume of the Medico-Chirurgical Transactions. Repair of injuries in paralyzed parts does not generally take place so readily or completely as in parts in which the nerves are in their normal condition. A case in support of this view is furnished by Mr. TRAVERS,* in which paraplegia was produced by fracture of the lumbar vertebræ, and in the same accident the humerus and tibia were fractured. The former in due time united, but the latter did not.

As undue prominence may by some be attached to the influence of the sympathetic system on nutrition, the following statement gives additional support to our position : " The defect of nutrition which ensues after lesion of the spinal cord alone, the sympathetic nerves being uninjured, and the general atrophy which sometimes occurs in consequence of diseases of the brain, seems to prove the influence of the cerebro-spinal system."†

Having considered some of the more marked effects of deficient nerve power on nutrition, and that alcohol, by interfering with the nutrition of the nervous system, to a certain extent causes these damaging effects, thereby accounting in part, it would seem, for retardation or partial

---

* Travers' Further Inquiry Concerning Constitutional Irritation, p. 436.
† Kirke's Manual of Physiology, p. 254.

arrest of *constructive* metamorphosis of tissue, we will now speak of some of the

SUPPOSED USES OF ALCOHOL

in the treatment of consumption. Besides being a retarder of tissue metamorphosis, which we have already considered, Prof. HENRY HARTSHORNE, of Philadelphia, in his valuable Essentials of Practical Medicine, while differing with us in opinion on this subject, says that "alcohol is useful— 1. By its direct excitant supporting power. 2. By aiding the enfeebled stomach to digest a larger supply of food." While this is the prevailing opinion of medical men, and therefore generally endorsed by the world at large, my own experience and investigations lead me to the conclusion that the following statements from a few of the most eminent authorities are nearest correct. In regard to the

TRANSIENTNESS OF THE EFFECTS OF STIMULANTS

Prof. STILLÉ says : "It is important to observe that by a law of the human economy the repeated impressions of a stimulus produce progressively feebler results. . . . All our senses are, to use the common and expressive term, blunted by the repetition of the same impressions upon them. [Illustrations of this are afforded in the fact that THEODORE HOOK and CHARLES LAMB grinned themselves into melancholy. Clowns are apt to be hypochondriac.

Hence the probable cause of the hypochondriasis of the man, who, upon consulting ABERNATHY, and being advised, as a remedy, to witness the performance of a great comedian who was playing at a neighboring theatre, replied, 'Alas! I am the great comedian.'] Every organ gradually becomes insensible to operations which at first may powerfully have excited it; even the affections lose their freshness, and the passions their fire; there is, in fact, nothing but pure intelligence which appears permanently and almost without limit to have its powers and susceptibilities increased by exercise. . . . Hence it is that not only stimuli which produce a local impression exclusively or chiefly, but those also which . . . are general and diffusible in their operation tend, by degrees, to exhaust the susceptibility of the system to their influence."*

The two propositions of Dr. HARTSHORNE, previously mentioned, regarding the stimulating value of alcohol to both the stomach and system at large, will, we believe, be seen to be fallacious when we consider the following statements: " A glass of malt liquor, or a small quantity of spirits, repeated three or four times a day, is found to increase the bodily vigor for a time; and this increase is set down as so much positive gain, no account being taken of the subsequent depression, which is considered as ordinary fatigue."† And against the second proposition the same

---

* Stillé's Materia Medica, 3d ed., vol. i, p. 557.
† Carpenter's Prize Essay on Alcoholic Liquors, p. 85.

author says : " If the stomach be not an exception to the general law of the action of stimulants upon the animal body, we should expect . . . . that the result of the moderate use of alcoholic stimulants will manifest itself sooner or later in diminution of the digestive power. The earliest indication of this, in most instances, is the demand for the augmentation of the stimulus to produce the same result, the amount which was at first sufficient to whet the appetite and increase the digestive power, being no longer found adequate. If the demand be yielded, and the quantity of the stimulus be augmented, the original benefit seems for a time to be derived from it ; but after the stomach has become tolerant of the liquor, that which at first excited it to increased functional activity, does so no longer, and a further increase is called for, until what began in ' moderation ' ends in positive *excess*, with all its consequent evils."*

After discussing at length the various items of evidence for and against the employment of alcoholic stimulants when there is a " demand for extraordinary exertion," " deficiency of other adequate sustenance," or " deficiency of constitutional vigor" (and to the latter category of course belongs the disease under consideration), Dr. CARPENTER in conclusion says: " On the whole, then, we may conclude that in by far the greater number of cases falling under one or other of the above categories, the influence of the habitual use of alcoholic liquors, while it may seem tem

* Prize Essay on Alcoholic Liquors, p. 129.

porarily beneficial, is in the end rather pernicious than otherwise."*

In concluding his remarks on the

"USE OF ALCOHOL IN EXCEPTIONAL CASES,"

the same author says : "The writer thinks that physiology and experience alike sanction the conclusion that although there are states of the stomach in which the diminished appetite and digestive power prevent the reception of an adequate supply of aliment into the system, and in which the assistance of alcoholic liquors is temporarily beneficial, that assistance is rather a *palliative* than a *cure* of the condition which calls for it; and, if perseveringly had recourse to, is likely to induce a train of evils of its own; . . . so great, that recourse should never be had to them until every other more natural method of sustaining the vital powers has been tried without success."†

We infer that the stimulating effect of alcohol on the stomach, like that produced in other parts of the body, is purely local, and explain its *modus operandi* as increasing the peristaltic or muscular action of the stomach, just as friction applied to the inner surface of the womb will stimulate that organ to post partum contraction, thereby promoting the comminution and timely propulsion of its contents, thus preventing the sense of weight or fullness

* Prize Essay on Alcoholic Liquors, p. 150.
† Ibid. pp. 159 and 160.

experienced at the epigastrium when the stomach remains unemptied an unusual length of time after ingestion. Hence we see why alcoholic stimulants are *apparently* useful in atony of the stomach. But as alcohol is directly destructive of pepsin, the most important property of the gastric juice, we fear that the increased facility of digestion is rather apparent than real. The chemical incompatibility of alcohol with pepsin is clearly shown in the fact that alcohol added to a solution of pepsin procured by digesting portions of the mucous membrane of the stomach in cold water after they have been macerated for some time in water at a temperature between 80° and 100° Fah., precipitates the pepsin in grayish-white flocculi.

Moreover, it has been the doom of the wine of pepsin to meet with but very little if any favor from those who have employed it; and Dr. J. S. UNZICKER, of Cincinnati, in a very interesting report to the Academy of Medicine, after having evidently given the subject a thorough investigation, says : " No wonder that so many observant physicians have always contended there was no therapeutic value in the wine of pepsin. Their conclusions were right, for Mr. EMIL SCHEFFER, a pharmaceutical chemist of Louisville, Ky., has clearly proven that the alcohol contained in the wine destroyed the pepsin. Consequently no effects can be expected from a solution of pepsin in a solvent containing alcohol."*

* *Philadelphia Medical and Surgical Reporter*, 1870, p. 264.

Then we can readily appreciate the correctness of the heretofore generally discredited statement of Prof. R. D. MUSSEY, viz.: "How wide from the truth is the notion that spirit aids the stomach in the process of digestion," which is further supported by the experiments of Dr. BEDDOES who observed that animals to whom he had given alcoholic stimulants along with their food, had digested nearly one-half less than other like animals to whom none had been given.*

The only advantage, then, that can be claimed for alcohol to the stomach in digestion is, that it promotes attenuation and propulsion of the food in cases in which the enfeebled stomach is unable to do this unassisted; and in doing so relieves the peculiar oppression experienced at the epigastrium in such cases. In thoroughly comminuting the food, of course the absorption of its nutritive constituents will be very much favored; but as the most important step in the process of digestion, viz., that of converting the albuminous constituents of the food into albuminose is interfered with by the destructive action of alcohol on pepsin, it is obvious that the pabulum formed when alcohol is ingested, is by no means adequate to *healthy* nutrition, as is shown in the unsoundness or low vitality of the tissues of persons (see previous remarks concerning "ballasters, brewers' draymen, coal-heavers," etc.) habituated to the

* See Mussey's Prize Essay on Ardent Spirits, p. 28.

use of alcoholic stimulants, which we believe is certainly a consequence of the imperfect digestion just described, as it also is of the deficient excretion which invariably attends the use of alcoholic liquors.   I prefer, then, with Dr. CAR-PENTER, not to employ these agents "until every other more natural method of treatment has been tried without success;" and as the reader will probably inquire, How is this atony of the stomach, with its imperfect performance of function and unpleasant sensations to be remedied ? I will state that for the atony of stomach I use those agents known as bitter tonics,—sulphate of quinine in solution with tincture of chloride of iron, or infusions of those agents, and rarely their tinctures, — but more frequently than either, the sulphate of quinine.   While these are tonics, they are also stomachics, and by administering them a short time (half or three-quarters of an hour) before eat-ing, they gradually tend to remedy the atonic condition referred to, while the oppression and imperfect action of the stomach is still further remedied by a combination of subnitrate of bismuth and BOUDAULT'S pepsin adminis-tered immediately after eating (three times a day), fol-lowed with thirty to forty drops of dilute nitric acid, thirty to forty minutes after administering the bismuth and pep-sin.   I would also state that I discontinue the bismuth (but not always the pepsin), as soon as the condition in question subsides.

Let us consider next the

EFFECTS OF ALCOHOL ON INFLAMMATION.

Inflammation, it is well known, is the direct source of mischief in tuberculosis. It is this, indeed, upon which its fatality depends; for the occurrence of ordinary tubercular deposition never proves fatal without the supervention of inflammation. It has recently been assumed that alcohol is an antiphlogistic, and this, if true, naturally enough adds to the category of supposed uses of that agent in the treatment of consumption. This extravagant assertion, however, is not suggestive to us of thoroughness of research or accuracy of observation. Our position on this point, as will presently be seen, is that alcoholic, among other forms of stimulation, cannot be produced without irritation,—the kind or degree of irritation differing, of course, according to the peculiar impression to be made upon the nervous centres through the medium of the senses,—and I now make the proposition, without, I believe, the risk of successful contradiction, that irritation, whether it be local or constitutional, superficial or deep seated, is nothing more nor less than absolute stimulation to the parts to which it is applied, and our position is supported not only by facts, but by the phraseology itself. The reader may ask, How do we explain this? When a goad or spur (which by WEBSTER is defined as a stimulant for this purpose) is thrust into the flank of the jaded roadster, he becomes irritated, and in consequence of that irritation is stimulated to increased exertion. And when men or the lower animals are mentally irritated by insult or injury, we notice an exaltation of their various faculties, especially that of pugnacity, so that they are enabled to commit acts of violence that in their normal state would be impossible. Again, animals of every grade and variety are by nature endowed with certain obvious means of self-defence—hence arises the old adage, "self-protection is the first law of nature." So these animals, when interfered with, defend themselves by biting, kicking, stinging, running, swimming, or flying away, or otherwise, according to their respective means of self-protection. And even in different organs or parts of the body,—indeed in *all parts* of the body,—we notice this faculty to be a prominent characteristic; as the contraction of the circular fibres of the iris upon the admission and by the action of light upon the retina, and the complete closure of the lids in keratitis —the causation of emesis and diarrhœa by the action and for the expulsion of irritating ingesta,—the increased mucus and lachrymal secretion for the removal of irritants or stimulating applications from the conjunctiva,—the augmentation of vital activity evinced by the inflammatory action and consequent suppuration or festering occasioned by the presence and for the removal of foreign bodies from various parts of the organism, all go to confirm us in the belief that irritation *is* stimulation, and that the local stimulation due to the application of rubefacients and epispastics is but an effort of nature to remove *from* the offending material,—the complete effect of which, when allowed to remain, is comparable to the injury or destruction of a small animal by a larger one whose violence it was unable to resist.

We would suggest, therefore, that defining or considering irritation as always being excessive stimulation of a part is not legitimate, because irritation (of course we have no reference to the painful depression which is the ultimate result of the immediate effects of the stimulus) is necessarily initiatory to stimulation; and that excessive local stimulation usually defined as irritation is only analogous to the excessive or toxical effects of a general stimulant. Let us now turn to the

MODUS OPERANDI OF ALCOHOL

as a general stimulant. We have already adverted to the fact that it enters the current of the circulation unchanged in its chemical composition. In common with other general stimulants (cantharides, mustard, ammonia, arnica, camphor, creasote, turpentine, toxicodendron, calor, galvanism, friction, etc.) when applied externally, it produces local stimulation identical with the effects of other rubefacients and epispastics; and if its application is continued, it excites permanent redness and even inflammation. Of course we cannot, then, do otherwise than suppose that when it comes in direct contact with the deep-seated tissues, which are much more delicate in their nature, and through which it has to pass in producing its constitutional effects, owing to their delicacy of structure, its local effect on those tissues will be correspondingly increased. And as local stimulation or irritation is always effected upon the sensitive nervous filaments of the part to which the stimulus or irritant is applied, exciting it to increased nervous, and therefore to augmented vascular and functional activity, and especially as, in the instance under consideration, it not only comes in direct contact with the nervous filaments of the vessels, but flows through the nervous centres themselves, it seems that this, notwithstanding its "special affinity for nervous substance," before referred to (which most probably explains the cause of the cerebral symptoms peculiar to and consequent upon its more marked poisonous effects on the brain), is a reasonable explanation of the *modus operandi* of alcohol as a general stimulant.

Having considered what we conceive to be its physiological *modus operandi*, it is not difficult for us to understand

HOW ALCOHOL DOES POSITIVE DAMAGE

to the lungs by aggravating, if not by causing their inflammation. The correctness of our hypothesis finds support

from no smaller authorities than TROUSSEAU, the great
French physician, and Dr. LANCEREAUX, of Paris. The
latter gentleman has pointed out the frequent occurrence
of inflammation of the vena porta, accompanied by pseudo-
membranous exudation in persons addicted to the habitual
use of alcoholic liquors; and in the same class of subjects
"there exists," he says, "a form of arteritis which is cha-
racterized anatomically by membranous formations on the
interior of the vessels. This form of arteritis, which I
have always met with in the pulmonary artery, may determine to a great extent, and in a manner altogether mechanical, coagulation of the blood, leading to obstruction of the
vessel and death. The frequency with which it is met in
drunkards, does not seem fortuitous; and there is every
reason to believe that it owes its origin to the abuse of
alcoholic drinks."*

M. TROUSSEAU on this point says, that "the alcohol alters
the condition of the walls of the pulmonary artery, and
consecutively the tissue of the lungs, just as it alters the
state of the parietes of the vena porta." "You can well
understand that it is impossible for the lungs, through the
medium of the pulmonary artery, to remain constantly in
contact with the alcoholic substance, without their delicate
tissue being injured. This is in reality what does occur.
In drunkards, every variety of pulmonary lesion is met
with, from congestion to inflammation and tubercle."

* Lancereaux:—*Gazette Medicale*, Paris, 1862.

"*Pulmonary congestion* is the most frequent of these lesions, for it is necessarily the first stage of all the others. . . . . . The congestion is all the more natural, that a portion of the absorbed alcohol traverses the pulmonary tissue that it may be eliminated during expiration, and that in doing so, it must necessarily irritate that tissue." "Pneumonia, likewise, is the consequence of the lung being thus impregnated with alcohol: . . . . for all these reasons, it can be understood that *under the influence of a predisposition or weakness, on the one hand,* [italics ours] *and of constant irritation of the lung on the other, tubercle becomes developed.*"* Alluding to a case of "hemorrhagic meningitis," TROUSSEAU says: "The alcoholic impregnation of the brain caused meningitis." "Throughout the entire arterial system, traces are to be found of the ravages committed by the passage and contact of alcohol." "Alcohol exercises a similar action upon every part of the organism."†

Add to the foregoing statements the weighty authority of Dr. CARPENTER and Prof. R. D. MUSSEY, and we will, as we believe, have made out a strong case. "It very frequently happens that the liver is the part in which a disposition to torpidity of the circulation exists; and congestion of its portal system of vessels must stagnate the whole of the circulation through the chylopoietic viscera,

* Trousseau's Clinical Medicine, vol. iii, pp. 436 and 437.
† Ibid. p. 441.

from which the blood of that system is derived. Any disposition to local congestion must operate with increased
force in producing general irregularity of the circulation ;
. . . and as hepatic and abdominal congestions are among
the ordinary results of excess in the use of alcoholic liquors,
it cannot be doubted but that even their *moderate* employment must aggravate any tendency to derangement of the
circulation when it already exists."* Prof. MUSSEY says :
" In *inflammations*, whether deep seated or superficial, the
vascular and nervous irritations are usually observed to be
increased by the use of alcoholic liquors."† Then,

OUR CONCLUSIONS

are, that as alcohol enters the current of the circulation
unchanged in its chemical composition, by its chemical
affinity for and action upon the albumen and red corpuscles of the blood, it prevents the elaboration of the plasma
and thereby seriously interferes with healthy nutrition ;
and that, by the peculiar way in which it acts as a retarder
of the retrograde metamorphosis of tissue, it interferes with
excretion, occasioning retention of effete matter, especially
carbon (which we believe to be unquestionably as detrimen-
tal to the normal performance of the various physiological
functions of the body as breathing an atmosphere abounding

* Carpenter's Prize Essay on Alcoholic Liquors, pp. 133 and 134.
† Prize Essay on Ardent Spirits, p. 52.

6

in carbonic acid with a consequent deficiency of oxygen), which should and would normally be eliminated; that owing to its special modification of the nutrition of the nervous substance, it is, as Prof. CHAMBERS, of London, says, " an arrester of nerve life, and consequently a controller of nervous action on the rest of the frame." This being the case, its indispensable influence on the nutrition and various vital processes of the body is materially interfered with, thus accounting in part, we believe, for its effects as a retarder of *con*structive metamorphosis of tissue; and that fatty degeneration of the liver, as TROUSSEAU wisely remarks, " is almost invariably met with in alcoholic drinkers," as it also is in the majority of cases of advanced consumption, making it reasonable to conclude that the development of this dreadful complication of the disease will be very much favored by the ingestion of alcoholic liquors, and that its fancied aid to digestion is *apparent* and *not* real, but that, on the other hand, on account of its destructive influence on pepsin,—the active principle of the gastric juice,—it renders digestion all the more imperfect, thus rendering bloodmaking and nutrition necessarily deficient, setting an impassable barrier to increase of strength and vigor; and that, according to the hypothesis upon which we explain the physiological *modus operandi* of alcoholic stimulants, and the excellent as well as eminent authorities by whom we are supported, inflammation,—the peculiar pathological process upon which the destruction of the lungs depends,— is always aggravated, if not frequently developed, by the action of alcohol upon them. For all these reasons, except in cases of extreme exhaustion, alcohol is not, under any circumstance, the consumptive's friend, but, indeed, is his meretricious and stealthy assassin.

INDEX.

Acherly, Dr., on nitric acid in whooping cough, 29.
Alcohol in consumption, 53.
    effects of, on tissues and fluids of the body, 53.
        albumen of blood, 54–56.
        red corpuscles of blood, 57.
        inflammation, 75.
        nutrition of nervous system, 63.
      in exciting nervous centres, 63,
    in the circulation, 55.
        ventricles of the brain, 55.
        blood, 55.
    as a retarder of *constructive* tissue metamorphosis, 59–61.
         destructive tissue metamorphosis, 59.
    darkens arterial blood, 57.
    an arrester of nerve life, 65.
    a cause of amblyopia, 66.
    agents used instead of, 74.
    damaging to the lungs, 78.
    destructive to pepsin, 72.
    delirium tremens produced by, 64.
    insanity produced by, 64.
        how produced by, 65.

(85)

Alcohol, modus operandi of, 77.

    supposed uses of, 68.

    on the use of, in exceptional cases, 71.

Amblyopia caused by alcoholic drinks, 66.

Arnoldi, Dr., on the value of nitric acid in whooping cough, 28.

Arterial blood, venous condition of, caused by alcohol, 58.

Author's conclusions, 81.

Bartholow, Prof. Roberts, on nitric acid in indigestion, 31.

Baumes on phosphoric acid in tuberculosis, 12.

Bennett, Prof. J. H., on calcareous deposits, 15.

Bennett, Dr. J. R., on phosphates in tuberculosis, 10.

Blood, effects of deficient plasticity of, 61.

Bouchardat, experiments of, 59.

Cases, 36–39.

    remarks on, 40–52.

Chapman on nitric acid in impetigo and scrofulous sores, 30.

Churchill, Dr., on phosphates in tuberculosis, 10.

Consumption, absence of, in Sologne, 12.

        alcohol in, 53,

        bad effects of hard water in, 12.

        causes of, 21.

        condition of plasma in, 19.

        effects of insufficient or improper diet in, 24.

        fatty liver in, 20.

            frequency of, 20.

        fresh air in, 24, 25.

        how produced by bad air and bad food, 25.

            chronic pneumonia, 26.

        lime in, 12.

        nitric and muriatic acids in, 28.

Consumption, pathology of, 9.

predisposition to, 21

how acquired, 24.

treatment of, 28.

Cotton, Dr., on phosphates in tuberculosis, 10.

Cretaceous tubercles, 13.

Davis, Prof. N. S., on alcohol in the current of the circulation, 55.

Duroy on alcohol in the current of the circulation, 55.

Elstun, Dr. W. J., on digestive assimilation of medicines, 33.

Freund, of Bresleau, on ossification in tuberculosis, 11.

Frick, Dr., on excess of lime in the blood of consumptives, 12.

Galezowski, M., on alcoholic amblyopia, 66.

Gibb on nitric acid in whooping cough, 29.

Glover, Dr., on nitric acid in chronic bronchitis, 29.

Graves on alcohol in the blood, 55.

Gray tubercles, 13.

consistency of, 13.

size of, 13.

Hartshorne, Prof. Henry, on phosphates in tuberculosis, 10.

hard water in tuberculosis, 12.

Heberden, Dr., on hard water in tuberculosis, 12.

lime in tuberculosis, 12.

Hemorrhage of the lungs, prescription for, 48.

Lactucarium, syrup of, 45.

Lallemand, M. M., on alcohol in the current of circulation, 55.

Lancereaux, Dr., on *alcoholic* arteritis, 79.

Lawson, Prof. L. M., on cretaceous tubercles, 13.

Lawson, Prof. L. M., on gray tubercles, 13.

                    phosphates in tuberculosis, 10.

Lungs, destruction of, 18.

            by caseous infiltration, rare, 27.

Maring, Rudolph, on alcohol in the current of circulation, 55.

Medicine, digestive assimilation of, 33.

Menelly, Dr., on nitric acid in whooping cough, 29.

Muriatic acid, properties of, 32.

                mode of administering, 35.

Mussey, Dr., on alcohol in the blood, 55.

Nervous system, influence of, on nutrition, 66.

                          examples where deficient, 66, 67.

Niemeyer on ossification in tuberculosis, 11.

Nitric acid, mode of administering, 34.

          in syphilis, 29.

             chronic affections of the liver, 29.

             augmenting muscular substance and strength, 31.

             dissolving phosphatic gravel, 31.

             healing phagadenic and flabby ulcers, 31.

             passive hemorrhage, 31.

          as an antiphosphatic, 31.

Nitrogenized food, 32.

                 in consumption, 32.

Noble, Dr., on nitric acid in whooping cough, 29.

Nutrition, influence of nervous system on, 66.

            as influenced by alcoholic drinks, 61–64.

Percy, Dr. John, experiments of, with alcohol, 55.

Perrin, experiments of, with alcohol, 55.

Phosphates a cause of tubercle, 9.

             inorganic element of tubercle, 9.

Phosphates in food, 11.

in tuberculosis, 10.

Plasma a deutoxide of proteine, 26–56.

Prout, Dr., experiments of, with alcohol, 59.

Prunus virginiana, syrup of, 45.

Pulmonary congestion caused by alcohol, 80.

Quain, Dr., on phosphates in tuberculosis, 10.

Royer on nitric acid in impetigo and scrofulous sores, 30.

Red corpuscles, function of, 57.

Richardson, Dr. B. W., on hard water in consumption, 12.

Stillé, Prof. Alfred, on nitric acid in the hoarseness of singers, 29.

transientness of the effects of stimulants, 68.

Stimulants, transientness of effects of, 68.

Stone, Dr. W., on phosphates in tuberculosis, 10.

Taylor, Mr. John, on phosphates in tuberculosis, 10.

Trousseau, M., on alcoholic arteritis, 79.

Tubercles, absorption of, 52.

analysis of, 9.

phosphates in, 9.

inorganic element of, 9.

deposition of, 15.

different forms of, 13–16.

transformation of, 16.

how accomplished, 16.

crude, source of, 16.

softening of, 17.

Tuberculization, modus operandi of, 17.

Tuberculosis, condition of urine in, 10.

origin of, 14.

Tuberculous matter, elimination of, 52.

                      mode of elimination of, 52.

Tuberculous elimination, nitric acid for, 52.

Wanner, M., on lime in tuberculosis, 12.

Watson, Sir Thos., on softening of tubercles, 17.

Whittaker, Prof. Jas. T., on ossification in tuberculosis, 11.

Williams, Dr. C. J. B., on nitric acid for fatty liver, 29.

Wood, Prof. Geo. B., on phosphates in tuberculosis, 10.

www.ingramcontent.com/pod-product-compliance
Lightning Source LLC
Chambersburg PA
CBHW031444270326
41930CB00007B/857